STOMACH ULCER TREATMENT

STOMACH ULCER TREATMENT, EASY DIET CARE AND HEAL REMEDY

Dr. David whitely

INTRODUCTION

Scientists have shown that since modern man migrated from Africa over 60,000 years ago, the common bacteria that causes the most painful stomach ulcers has been present in the human digestive system. They discovered that the genetic differences between human populations that developed as they disseminated from Eastern Africa over thousands of years are duplicated in H. pylori by comparing the DNA sequence patterns of humans and the Helicobacter pylori bacteria, which is now known to cause the majority of stomach ulcers.

Gastric ulcers and stomach ulcers are both painful sores in the stomach lining. Peptic ulcer illness includes conditions like stomach ulcers. Peptic ulcers are any ulcers that impact the small intestine and the stomach.

Reduced levels of the thick coating of mucus that shields your stomach from digestive fluids cause stomach ulcers to develop. This makes the stomach tissues eroded by the digestive acids, leading to an ulcer.

Although stomach ulcers are usually treatable, they can worsen if not treated properly.

Hyperacidity can also be confused with a straightforward stomachache. Therefore, paying attention to how frequently you have stomach pain is crucial and whether you also experience the following symptoms: bloating, burping, or a sour taste in your mouth. If untreated, persistent hyperacidity may result in ulcers or other problems.

While preventing causes of hyperacidity should be the priority, over-the-counter (OTC) remedies like antacids are popular because they instantly neutralize the stomach's acidity and raise its pH level. Relief from the antacid's effects may be felt immediately in the form of decreased stomach pain.

CHAPTER 1

WHAT IS STOMACH ULCER?

Gastric ulcers sometimes referred to as stomach ulcers, are lesions that form on the stomach's lining.

Duodenal ulcers are ulcers that can develop in the area of the intestine that is immediately after the stomach.

The symptoms of duodenal ulcers, also known as peptic ulcers, are the same as those of stomach ulcers, and their treatments are also the same.

HISTORY OF STOMACH ULCER

Scholars have long taken great satisfaction in their familiarity with works from earlier ages. For centuries, conventional education has been centered on ideas and writings that date back to ancient Greece. By the middle to end of the 20th century, this tradition was waning, coinciding with an enormous influx of new knowledge that made it impossible to keep up with what was known at the time and increased specialization. Pre-20th-century medical observations were largely ignored or forgotten. The development of electronic databases, which increased accessibility to recent material but did not index earlier literature, encouraged and abetted this tendency.

Significant changes in the clinical manifestations of H. pylori infection occurred in European countries and the

U.S in the latter 1/2 of the 19th century and the first half of the 20th century, including variations in the type and incidence of peptic ulcer disease and a decline in gastric cancer. These modifications were not widespread and were mainly restricted to today regarded as industrialized Western nations. Similar developments are also taking place in several Asian countries as they transition from developing to developed status, as will be detailed later.

Henriette-Anne, the daughter of King Charles I, passed away unexpectedly at the age of 26 in 1670, one day after expressing discomfort in her abdomen. An autopsy was conducted since poisoning was suspected, and the results showed peritonitis and a tiny hole in the stomach's anterior wall.

Edward Crisp documented the first 50 occurrences of peptic perforation in 1843, and he precisely defined its clinical features, saying: "The symptoms are so typical, I hardly believe it possible that anyone may fail to make the correct diagnosis." Crisp's observation that stomach perforations were filled by adhesions to the nearby viscera, preventing leaking from the stomach into the peritoneal cavity, gave rise to the fundamental concept for conservative treatment.

Every doctor, faced with an open duodenal ulcer of the stomach or intestine, must consider opening the abdomen, suturing the hole, and preventing a potential inflammation by careful cleansing of the abdominal cavity, according to Johan Mikulicz-Radecki (1850-1905), who is frequently cited as the first surgeon to close a perforated peptic ulcer by simple closure.

The 1946 introduction of the Taylor method of conservative management was based on the idea that efficient gastric decompression and continuous drainage would promote self-healing, leading to treatment with nasogastric aspiration, antibiotics, intravenous fluids, and currently H. pylori triple therapy.

By doing a gastro duodenogram, as Donovan indicated, patients likely to respond to conservative therapy can be chosen.

Today, surgery for peptic ulcer disease is only used to address complications like bleeding, perforation, etc. In some situations of peptic perforation, conservative treatment may be used. If laparotomy is required, simple closure is usually sufficient, and patients no longer need to have definitive ulcer surgery. [10] Centers with laparoscopy equipment and the necessary experience perform laparoscopic perforation closure.

UNDERSTANDING YOUR DIGESTION AND GUT

The G.I., often known as the digestive tract and the liver, pancreas, and gallbladder, make up the digestive system. A long, twisted tube from the mouth to the anus is the G.I. tract, which comprises several hollow organs. The hollow organs that include the gastrointestinal tract (G.I. tract) are the mouth, esophagus, stomach, small intestine, large intestine, and anus. The liver, pancreas, and gallbladder are referred to as the solid organs of the digestive system.

Three sections make up the small intestine. The duodenum is the name of the first section. The ileum is at the end, while the jejunum is in the middle. The cecum, colon, rectum, and appendix are all parts of the large intestine. A finger-shaped pouch connected to the cecum is the appendix. The beginning of the big intestine is the cecum. The colon follows. The big intestine empties into the rectum.

Each component of the digestive system either breaks down food and drink into smaller pieces, moves food and liquid through the GI tract, or does both. The human body can absorb and transport nutrients from food once it has been cut into smaller particles. The waste products of digestion turn into fesses due to the large intestine absorbing water. Nerves and hormones regulate the digestive process.

Peristalsis is the physiological process through which food passes through the GI tract. The GI tract's significant, hollow organs are covered in a layer of muscle that allows the walls to move. The motion mixes the contents of each organ as it forces food and liquid through the GI tract. While the muscle in front of the meal relaxes to allow the food to travel, the muscle behind it contracts to force the food forward.

The digestive system starts in the mouth. In actual sense, digestion begins even before you take a meal. The salivary glands start to work as soon as you see the meal or perceive the aroma. When you start eating, you chew your food to break it up into bite-sized pieces that are easier to digest. Your saliva begins to break down the meal into a form your body can absorb and utilize. Your tongue help move the food from your mouth into your throat and esophagus as you swallow.

The esophagus is in your throat next to your trachea, where food travels from the mouth (windpipe). To prevent choking, a little flap covering your windpipe known as the epiglottis is present when you swallow. Peristalsis, a series of esophageal muscular contractions, is the process by which food enters your stomach.

The lower esophageal sphincter, a ring-shaped muscle at the bottom of your esophagus, must first loosen to allow food to enter. The sphincter then tightens, stopping the stomach contents from returning to the esophagus. (If it doesn't, you could have acid reflux or heartburn when these substances flow back into the esophagus.)

A hollow organ, the stomach acts as a "container" for food while it is processed by stomach enzymes. These enzymes continue preparing the meal so that it may be ingested. Powerful acids and strong enzymes released by stomach lining cells carry out the breakdown process. Once properly digested, the stomach's contents are expelled into the small intestine.

The duodenum, jejunum, and ileum comprise the small intestine. This muscular tube measuring 22 feet in length is used to break down food utilizing pancreatic enzymes and bile from the liver. Food movement through this organ, when mixed with pancreatic and liver juices during peristalsis, is another function of this organ.

The small intestine's first section is called the duodenum. It is primarily to blame for the ongoing breakdown process. The bottom portions of the gut, the jejunum, and ileum, are mainly responsible for nutrient absorption into the bloodstream.

After passing through the small intestine, the contents change from semi-solid to liquid. The change in consistency is caused by a combination of water, bile, enzymes, and mucus. The liquid remaining from the meal passes through the small intestine after the nutrients have been absorbed and before entering the large intestine (colon).

Digestive enzymes are sent from the pancreas into the duodenum where they break down protein, lipids, and carbohydrates. In addition, the pancreas makes and releases insulin directly into the blood. Insulin is mostly used by your body to metabolize sugar.

Although the liver serves a number of roles in the digestive system, processing nutrients taken through the small intestine is its primary duty. The small intestine receives bile from the liver, which helps with vitamin absorption and the breakdown of fat.

The liver serves as the body's chemical "factory." It uses the fundamental components the gut absorbs to produce all the many chemicals your body needs to function.

Additionally, the liver detoxifies potentially dangerous substances. Numerous medications that can be hazardous to your body are broken down and secreted by it.

Bile from the liver is stored in the gallbladder before being released into the duodenum of the small intestine to help absorb and digest lipids.

The colon is in charge of regulating waste to make it simple and convenient to empty your bowels. The muscular tube that joins the small intestine to the rectum is 6 feet long.

The cecum, the ascending colon (right), the transverse colon (across), the descending colon (left), and the sigmoid colon, which joins to the rectum, make up the colon.

By use of peristalsis, feces, or waste from the digestive process, is transferred through the colon, first in a liquid state and then in a solid form. Water is expelled from the stool as it moves through the colon. The stool is kept in the sigmoid (S-shaped) colon until it is emptied into the rectum once or twice daily during a "mass movement.

Stool typically passes through the colon for about 36 hours or such. Bacteria and food particles make up the majority of the stool itself. These "good" bacteria carry out a variety of practical tasks, including producing different vitamins, processing food scraps and waste, and guarding against harmful bacteria. The descending colon releases its contents into the rectum to start the elimination process when it is full of stool, also known as feces (a bowel movement).

The 8-inch-long, straight chamber is known as the rectum and joins the colon to the anus. The rectum's duties include:

- Collecting stool from the colon.
- Alerting you to the presence of stool.
- Holding the stool until evacuation occurs.

When something (such as gas or excrement) reaches the rectum, sensors notify the brain. The decision to remove the rectal contents is then made by the brain.

Sphincters open if they can, and the rectum contracts to push the contents out. The sphincter contracts and the rectum adapts, momentarily eliminating the feeling, if the contents cannot be expelled.

The anus is the last part of the digestive system. A 2-inch canal houses the two anal sphincters and the pelvic floor muscles (internal and external). The upper anus lining can be used to feel the rectus contents. You can see if the contents are in a liquid, gas, or solid condition.

Sphincter muscles vital for controlling feces are located all around the anus. To prevent wastes from going out when it shouldn't, the pelvic floor muscle angles the rectum and the anus. The internal sphincter is constantly tight except when stool enters the rectum. When we are asleep or ignorant of the presence of stool, this maintains our continent (prevents us from pooping involuntarily).

When we need to use the restroom, we rely on our external sphincter to contain the stool until we arrive at the toilet, which relaxes and lets the contents out.

MECHANISM OF STOMACH ULCER

In the United States, gastric ulcers are a prevalent clinical manifestation that frequently results in spending millions of dollars on medical care. They are larger than

5 mm in diameter and represent a breach in the mucosal barrier of the stomach lining that penetrates the muscularis mucosa. It's crucial to realize that this illness process can be both prevented and treated. Depending on the cause of the patient's stomach ulcer, numerous treatment options may be available. The body naturally shields the stomach mucosa from the potentially dangerous gastric lumen's acidic environment.

When these defenses are compromised, the stomach mucosa may undergo changes resulting in erosion and ulceration. Prostaglandins, mucus, growth factors, and proper blood flow protect the gastric mucosa. Smoking, hydrochloric acid, ischemia, NSAIDs, hypoxia, alcohol, and Helicobacter pylori infection are harmful factors of this barrier.

The two most frequent causes of stomach ulcers are gastric prostaglandin loss by non-steroidal anti-inflammatory drugs and Helicobacter pylori bacterium infection. Some of these are hypergastrinemia (Zollinger-Ellison syndrome), viral infections like CMV, chemotherapy, radiation, gastric outlet blockage, gastric infiltrative illnesses like malignancy, smoking, and Crohn's disease, the less frequent etiologies. All of these etiologies have one thing in common: they encourage the collapse of the mucosal barrier, exposing the gastric mucosa to the harmful effects of acid.

Let's start with Helicobacter pylori, which colonizes between 45 and 50 percent of the stomach mucosa globally. People get immunized against this bacterium at a young age, particularly in developing nations where the socioeconomic position is lower, and housing is more congested.

Due to the inflammatory reaction that these bacteria cause in the host, gastritis—a condition marked by epithelial damage and degeneration—occurs. Pan-gastritis frequently occurs in those who have this infection. As a result, the release of somatostatin from the antral region is impaired, which raises gastrin secretion and promotes more significant acid generation. Those patients whose bacterium has persisted in the antrum will eventually develop stomach ulcers.

The more proximal stomach body's parietal cells still have total production capacity, preventing the creation of ulcers there. Not all individuals with this infection experience symptoms; this depends on the virulence of the bacteria and other host risk factors. The development of cagA, which causes more significant cytokine cell death and mucosal injury, is a typical bacterial virulence factor.

The second most frequent cause generating stomach ulcers is NSAID medicines. When compared to persons who don't take these medications, patients who do have a relative risk of four stomach ulcers, NSAIDs can cause ulceration through a variety of different methods. When exposed to gastric acid, the medications themselves are weak acids. They persist in the epithelial cells and increase cellular permeability, which causes actual damage to the cells. The reduction in prostaglandin synthesis is the leading cause of NSAID-induced ulceration.

NSAIDs prevent the cyclooxygenase-1 enzyme from increasing prostaglandin synthesis, which promotes gastric bicarbonate secretion, the formation of mucus barriers, an increase in mucosal blood flow, and an expedited rate of epithelial cell restitution and repair following damage or cell death. NSAID drugs make the stomach mucosa susceptible to injury from pepsin and gastric acid. Overall, the decrease in gastric blood flow and the mild ischemia it generates in the stomach mucosa cause the most detrimental physiological damage.

The pathophysiology of gastric ulcer development mostly varies on the etiology, but they all result in the destruction or loss of the integrity of the stomach mucosa.

HEART BURN OR STOMACH ULCER SOME KEY DIFFERENCES

Heart burn

Heartburn is a burning sensation below your ribs, behind your breastbone, or in the middle of your chest. In addition to the tongue feeling bad, you could also feel it in your chest. Additionally, you can get chest pain when bending over or lying down. Have a burning, acidic, bitter, or salty sensation in your esophagus? Do you have trouble swallowing? Heartburn is, then.

Heartburn irritates the esophageal tube, which connects your neck and stomach. The culprits are the digestive fluids. Under the breastbone, the upper abdomen experiences burning as a result. Contrary to popular belief, heartburn has little to do with the heart. However some symptoms are similar to those of a heart attack or heart disease, others are not.

The main distinction between heartburn and ulcer is that an ulcer is a narrow burning sensation or abscess in the wall of your stomach or small intestine, the very first part of your intestinal wall, whereas heartburn happens when acid reflux rises into your esophagus, to cause a burning feeling (also known as acid indigestion) and a bad taste on the back of your tongue.

ULCER

Long-lasting or recurrent sores are known as ulcers. They can happen inside or outside your body and come in various sizes, shapes, and colors. They typically occur in places where topical medication cannot be used.

In most cases, the proximal portion of the small intestine's stomach mucosa exhibits it as an open wound. Letting stomach acids inside can breach the tissue's protective layer.

CHAPTER 2

STOMACH ULCER: CAUSES AND SYMPTOMS

What causes stomach ulcers?

H. pylori bacteria and a type of painkillers known as nonsteroidal anti-inflammatory medications are the two primary causes of stomach and small intestine ulcers (NSAIDs).

Excessive stomach acidity, often known as hyperacidity, and Zollinger-Ellison syndrome are less frequent causes of stomach ulcers.

Genetics, smoking, stress, and particular meals are just a few factors that might contribute to excess stomach acidity.

Stomach ulcers are a danger when using NSAIDs. Aspirin and ibuprofen are the two NSAIDs that are most often used.

If the medications are taken often for an extended period or in large quantities, the risk of ulcers increases.

The risk of stomach ulcers is higher with stronger NSAIDs, such as those prescribed than with over-the-counter NSAIDs.

When using painkillers, a person should carefully read the labels and get advice from a doctor or pharmacist. They might suggest acetaminophen as an alternative.

Several variables, including: an increase the possibility of getting a stomach ulcer.

Using steroids regularly, being hypercalcemic, having too much calcium in the blood, and drinking alcohol frequently.

People above sixty are more likely to get stomach ulcers. Although stomach ulcers can occur at any age, they are significantly less prevalent in young children. If their parents smoke, children are more in danger.

H. pylori infections are typical and typically harmless for most people.

However, it can occasionally result in duodenal or gastric ulcers (duodenal ulcer).

The reason some people are more affected than others is unclear.

SIGNS AND SYMPTOMS OF STOMACH ULCERS

The belly button and breastbone area will probably be painful or uncomfortable. This might increase when one is hungry, such as in between meals or at night. If you eat or take an antacid, the pain can disappear for a short period before coming back. The discomfort may come and go for several days or weeks, lasting only a few minutes or several hours.

Other signs can include:

- Bloated sensation

- Burping

- Having no appetite or losing weight

- Nausea

- Dark or bloody feces

- Vomiting

WHEN TO SEEK MEDICAL ADVICE

Although stomach ulcers can be treated, they should still

be regarded carefully. They're not a good indicator, even

if they don't result in symptoms. When you develop a

stomach ulcer, your body's natural stomach acid overpowers your stomach's barrier-protecting lining. It will only worsen if no action is taken to control the issue. Although lifestyle modifications may be helpful, the underlying problem must still be treated. It's most likely NSAID usage or widespread bacterial infection. The best medications for your illness might be recommended by your healthcare professional.

WHO IS MORE LIKELY TO DEVELOP ULCER

A peptic ulcer is more likely to form in people of any age who frequently take NSAIDs daily or many times per week. Aspirin and ibuprofen are painkillers known as

NSAIDs. Peptic ulcer disease can result from long-term NSAID use.

If you take NSAIDs, also known as NSAID-induced peptic ulcers, your risk of developing one increases.

Female, at least 70 years old, taking more than two NSAID types, or have taken NSAIDs frequently for a long time.

Have experienced a peptic ulcer in the past

Have two or more medical conditions or diseases and/or are taking additional medications, such as corticosteroids and bone-building medications.

Alcohol or smoking.

Infections with H. pylori affect between 30 and 40 percent of adults in the US. The disease typically remains latent or quiet without any signs or symptoms for years. Most people first get an H. pylori infection as children.

Adults with an H. pylori infection may develop a peptic ulcer, also known as an H. pylori-induced peptic ulcer. However, the majority of individuals with an H. pylori infection never get peptic ulcer disease. Children rarely get H. pylori-related stomach ulcers.

Spiral-shaped bacteria called H. pylori can harm the lining of your stomach and duodenum and lead to peptic ulcer disease. How H. pylori spread is a mystery to researchers. They believe the bacteria might spread by;

→ Unhealthy food

→ Unhygienic eating utensils and water

→ Body fluids and saliva of an infected person.

Since H. pylori have been discovered in some infected individuals' saliva, an infection can spread by direct contact with other bodily fluids or saliva.

The peptic ulcers that malignancies bring on Zollinger-Ellison syndrome (ZES) patients experience. Although anyone might develop ZES, it is uncommon and only affects one in every million individuals. However, ZES is more prevalent in men between 30 and 50. A kid is more likely to have Zollinger-Ellison syndrome if one of the parents has multiple endocrine neoplasia type 1.

CHAPTER 3

TYPES OF STOMACH ULCER

An ulcer is a sore that hurts, heals slowly, and occasionally reappears. There are often ulcers. The reasons behind their occurrence and the associated symptoms are often influenced by their underlying causes.

From the surface of your skin to the lining of your stomach, ulcers can develop anywhere on or in your body.

Ulcers occasionally go away on their own. To avoid significant consequences, they may also need medical care.

STOMACH ULCER/ PEPTIC ULCER

Peptic or stomach ulcers are ulcers that form in the lining of the small intestine or stomach. An imbalance of digestive fluids brings them on, frequently brought on by an H. Pylori infection or frequent anti-inflammatory drugs. Heartburn, stomach pain, nausea, weight loss, and other symptoms are some of the signs and symptoms of peptic ulcers. Medication provided by a gastroenterologist can effectively treat them.

DUODENAL ULCER

The upper small intestine is where duodenal ulcers, a type of peptic ulcer, develop. The most prevalent sign of a duodenal ulcer is a pain in the mid to upper stomach area, especially if the discomfort is worse when the stomach is empty or prevents one from having a good sleep mainly at night.

EPIGASTRIC ULCER/ OESOPHAGEAL ULCER

Ulcers that form inside the esophagus are referred to as esophageal ulcers. Usually, lifestyle and dietary modifications, together with specific drugs and other treatments, can treat these ulcers.

INDIGESTION HEARTBURN

When acids in the stomach rise into the esophagus, it causes heartburn, a painful ailment. Simply put, the lining of your esophagus lacks the same protective layers that allow your stomach to withstand digesting solid acids. As a result, heartburn is a persistent ache in your chest, and possibly your throat caused when acid runs up into your esophagus, a condition known as acid reflux.

Up to 20% of Americans experience heartburn on a weekly basis, making it a rather prevalent condition. Men and women, young and elderly, even infants and young children are affected.

Heartburn can linger for a short while or for several hours, and it frequently gets worse right after eating. Heartburn can prevent you from getting a good night's sleep in addition to being painful.

Why Do You Get Heartburn?

Many different factors can cause heartburn, but eating is the biggest offender. It can also be brought on by overeating or simply eating a large, heavy meal right before night. We're looking at you, greasy fries and spicy wings.

Alcoholic and carbonated beverages can also cause heartburn. Overweight people frequently experience heartburn. The pressure from even a few additional pounds might cause acid to back up into your esophagus and put a strain on your stomach.

Indigestion: What Is It?

The medical term for it is dyspepsia. However, you might call it an upset stomach, a stomachache, or even a bellyache. Whatever name you give it, indigestion is an unpleasant, occasionally excruciating sensation that usually occurs after or after eating.

In most situations, overeating, eating quickly, or consuming foods your body doesn't react well to—typically foods high in fat—causes indigestion. In addition to indigestion, chewing with your mouth open might cause it. Belching and bloating, two additional symptoms of indigestion, can be brought on by swallowing too much air when eating.

How Does Indigestion Start?

Your symptoms of indigestion may include abdominal discomfort, bloating (a feeling of fullness), gas and belching, nausea, vomiting, a "growling" stomach, acidic mouth taste, and even diarrhea. Stress usually worsens symptoms, although they typically pass within a few hours.

Acid reflux illness, pancreatic abnormalities, and other more severe chronic disorders, including ulcers, can all be associated with indigestion. Talk to your health care provider if the symptoms are severe or last for longer than two weeks.

PEPTIC AND GASTRIC ULCER

The tunica intima or inner surface of the stomach or small intestine can become inflamed with peptic ulcers when the digestive tract's acid attacks it. The acid can produce an uncomfortable open sore that could bleed.

A mucous layer covers the lining of your digestive tract, often buffering it against acid. However, you might get an ulcer if the acid content is raised or the mucus content is lowered.

DUODENAL ULCER

A type of ulcer that develops in the lining of the section of the small intestine right above the stomach is known as a duodenal ulcer (the duodenum). Gastric ulcer refers to an ulcer in the stomach's lining.

Non-ulcer Dyspepsia (Functional Dyspepsia), Stomach Ulcer (Gastric Ulcer), Acid Reflux, and Oesophagitis refer to distinct leaflets.

An infection with Helicobacter pylori typically leads to a duodenal ulcer (H. pylori). The ulcer will heal after a 4- to 8-week course of acid-suppressing medication. One week of two antibiotics and an acid-suppressing drug will typically successfully treat the H. pylori infection. This usually stops the ulcer from returning. Duodenal ulcers can occasionally be brought on by anti-inflammatory medications used to treat illnesses like arthritis. You might need long-term acid-suppressing medication to keep taking the anti-inflammatory prescription.

NAUSEA

Nausea is a feeling of nausea and the desire to vomit. The urge to hurl the stomach contents can be preceded by nausea. The disorder can frequently be avoided and has a wide range of reasons.

Causes of nausea

Numerous factors can trigger nausea. Some people have heightened sensitivity to sounds, smells, tastes, drugs, and the impacts of certain medical disorders. These are all possible sources of nausea.

When you eat, the contents of your stomach may reflux back up into your esophagus if you have heartburn or gastroesophageal reflux disease (GERD). This produces a scorching feeling that makes people feel nausea.

Viral or bacterial gastrointestinal problems can cause nausea. Food poisoning is a condition brought on by foodborne germs. Additionally, viral infections might make you sick.

Certain drugs, such as those used in cancer treatments like chemotherapy, might cause nausea or upset the stomach. Read the drug information for any new medicines you may take very carefully.

A rough trip in a car can cause motion sickness and seasickness. This movement may result in a misalignment of the signals from the senses to the brain, which could cause nausea, vertigo, or vomiting.

Foods that are hot or heavy in fat or, when consumed in excess, can upset the stomach and make you feel sick. Eating things to which you are allergic can make you sick as well.

Symptoms of nausea might be exacerbated by severe pain. This is valid for severe illnesses like pancreatitis, gallstones, and/or kidney stones.

Nausea may be exacerbated by ulcers or sores in the stomach or small intestinal lining. An ulcer might make you feel hot and nauseous right after eating.

Additionally, nausea can be a sign of a number of different medical disorders, such as:

→ Harmless recurrent positional vertigo (BPPV)

→ Hearing loss

→ Heart attack, intestinal obstruction, liver failure, meningitis, or liver cancer.

If heart attack symptoms accompany your nausea, get quick medical attention. Crushing chest pain, a severe headache, jaw discomfort, sweat, or pain in your left arm are all signs of a heart attack.

If you feel nausea, a bad headache, a stiff neck, trouble breathing, or confusion, you should also get emergency help. Seek medical attention if you think you may have consumed something harmful or feel dehydrated.

If nausea has prevented you from consuming food or liquids for longer than 12 hours, consult a doctor. You should also visit your doctor if your nausea does not go away after 24 hours of attempting over-the-counter remedies.

Always seek medical treatment if you believe you have a medical emergency.

The onset of nausea can be delayed by avoiding its causes. To avoid are the following:

→ Flashing lighting, which can cause migraines

→ Humidity and heat

→ Strong odors during maritime cruises, such as those from perfume and cooking

Motion sickness can also be avoided by taking scopolamine, an anti-nausea medicine, before traveling.

You can lessen nausea by changing your eating habits, such as eating small, frequent meals. Minimizing nausea can also be achieved by avoiding strenuous exercise after meals. Avoiding oily, hot, or spicy foods can also be beneficial.

Cereal, crackers, bread, gelatin, and broth are a few examples of foods that are less likely to make you feel queasy.

Most common types of ulcer

Peptic ulcer

A peptic ulcer is a lesion that appears when the lining of the digestive system becomes damaged by digestive juices. The stomach lining, duodenum, or lower section of the esophagus can all develop peptic ulcers. Weight loss, nausea, and indigestion-like pain are possible symptoms.

Facts on peptic ulcers

The digestive system might be affected anywhere by peptic ulcers.

Nausea and stomach pain, which can occasionally feel like indigestion, are symptoms.

Bacteria and specific types of medications are among the causes.

Proton pump inhibitors (PPIs) and antibiotics are used as treatments.

People frequently have peptic ulcers without exhibiting any symptoms at all. However, indigestion-like pain is among the most prevalent signs and symptoms of peptic ulcers.

The discomfort may appear anywhere from the belly button to the breastbone; it may be short or persist for several hours. Depending on where it is located, it is worse during sleep occasionally and more painful when the stomach is empty or shortly after eating. Eating particular foods may make it worse, while other foods may help.

Other signs comprise:

Eating food that comes back up after swallowing it and feeling sick after eating it

Decrease in appetite and weight.

Complications The risk of complications rises depending on whether the ulcer is treated or not. Possible complications include:

Inside bleeding

Internal bleeding can cause hemodynamic instability, a dangerous condition impacting several organs.

Scar tissue, pyloric stenosis, ongoing inflammation of the stomach or duodenum lining, and peritonitis, in which the ulcer perforate through the wall of the small intestine or stomach

Stomach ulcers can come back. A first ulcer raises the likelihood of later acquiring another one.

GASTRIC ULCER

The stomach lining or small intestine can become infected with sores called stomach ulcers. They develop as a result of the stomach's protecting mucus being ineffective.

To aid in food digestion and ward off pathogens, the stomach creates a powerful acid. The stomach also secretes a thick coating of mucus to cover body tissues to shield them from this acid.

Acid can harm the stomach tissue, leading to ulcers if the mucus layer is worn down and no longer functions properly.

According to statistics from Western nations, 1 in 10 persons may experience a stomach or small intestine ulcer at some point in their lives.

Indigestion, often known as dyspepsia, is a typical symptom of a stomach ulcer.

Stomach pain or discomfort is a symptom of indigestion. Heartburn, which can also happen simultaneously as this symptom, can be confused for it.

Heartburn may be brought on by gastroesophageal reflux disease or acid reflux. People will feel it in the bottom of their chest because it happens a little higher up from the stomach.

Heartburn symptoms tend to be more specific than stomach ulcer symptoms, yet symptoms might still be hazy.

Additionally, an ulcer frequently causes a dull or burning discomfort in the middle of the abdomen. The pain is occasionally described as biting or gnawing. Some people might mention feeling hungry.

Although stomach ulcers are usually treatable, they can have severe consequences if they are not treated.

Additional signs include:

Unaccounted-for weight loss

Nauseous and dizzy

Not eating due to issues such as pain, bloating, burping, and a feeling of fullness. Consuming the recommended amount of fluids for red or tarry stools

Chest pain exhaustion

Eating, drinking, or using antacids may also be effective ways for people to manage their pain.

Some stomach ulcers are not discovered since they don't cause the typical indigestion-type discomfort. These ulcers are less frequent, and doctors only treat them after they begin bleeding.

Stomach wall holes can develop as a result of some ulcers. This severe illness, which doctors refer to as perforation,

In addition to changing over time, stomach ulcer symptoms might be challenging to identify.

Diet

Dietary modifications can aid in preventing the emergence of stomach ulcers.

Those who are susceptible to stomach ulcers should consume more of the following nutrients:

Eating various fruits and vegetables is essential for maintaining a healthy lining of the digestive tract. These foods have cytoprotective and anti-inflammatory qualities, are high in antioxidants, reduce acid release, and are rich in antioxidants. These are all crucial elements for preventing and treating ulcers, according to a 2017 study.

Diets rich in soluble dietary fiber lower the likelihood of stomach ulcers forming.

Helicobacter pylori (H. pylori) infections can be lessened by eating foods with live bacteria, such as probiotic yogurt. Probiotics have been demonstrated to somewhat reduce the impact of antibiotic side effects and gastrointestinal symptoms.

Vitamin C: When consumed at microscopic levels over an extended period, this potent antioxidant may help eradicate H. pylori. Vitamin C is abundant in vegetables, fruits, and legumes like oranges and tomatoes.

Avoiding substances that increase stomach acid production, such as alcohol and coffee, can also help lower the risk. Stomach ulcers may result from this, in turn.

DUODENAL ULCER

A duodenal ulcer is a lesion that develops in the duodenum's lining. The first section of your small intestine, or duodenum, is where food passes initially after leaving your stomach in your digestive system.

Both the duodenum and the stomach are susceptible to ulcers. Peptic ulcers include both duodenal and stomach ulcers. You have "peptic ulcer disease" if you have either of these symptoms.

What causes duodenal ulcers?

A potent acid produced by your stomach aids in food digestion and kills microorganisms. The cells of the stomach and duodenum create a mucus barrier around themselves to shield them from this acid. An ulcer may develop if this barrier is compromised.

Infection with the bacteria Helicobacter pylori, or H. pylori, is the principal contributor to this harm. An ulcer may develop due to the bacteria irritating the duodenal lining.

Some drugs, especially anti-inflammatory ones like ibuprofen and aspirin, can result in a duodenal ulcer.

Rarely, other medications or other issues could lead to an ulcer.

Smoking, excessive alcohol consumption, and stress may increase your risk of developing a duodenal ulcer, but these factors are not as significant as H. pylori infection.

If H pylori cause your ulcer, the usual treatment is 'triple therapy. This involves taking two antibiotics to kill the bacteria and medicine to reduce the amount of acid your stomach makes.

Suppose you don't have an H. pylori infection and have been using anti-inflammatory drugs. In that case, you will need to stop taking them (if possible) and start taking medication to reduce acid production in your stomach.

Drinking less alcohol, Taking antacids, and quitting smoking.

ESOPHAGEAL ULCER

The esophageal lining which is, the tube that connects the throat to the stomach, is where an esophageal ulcer, a specific type of peptic ulcer, develops.

When the layer of mucus that coats and shields the gastrointestinal tract wear away, esophageal ulcers develop.

This enables gut wall irritation brought on by stomach acid and other gastric secretions to result in ulceration.

Exposure to stomach acid: This results in long-term esophageal edema and irritation, which promotes the growth of ulcers. People with various gastrointestinal problems are more likely to experience stomach acid exposure. These can include severe heartburn and GERD, often known as gastrointestinal reflux disease or Hiatal hernias.

Drugs: Several medications, including aspirin, ibuprofen, bisphosphonates, and some antibiotics, can result in esophagitis, esophageal inflammation, and esophageal ulcers.

Infection: Although esophageal ulcers brought on by infections are uncommon, they have been linked to herpes, the human papillomavirus (HPV), and the fungus known as candida.

Esophageal ulcers may develop as a result of consuming a caustic chemical. Most victims of this damage are youngsters, although it can also happen to adults with psychosis, suicidal thoughts, or alcohol abuse problems.

BLEEDING ULCER

Digestive tract sores called peptic ulcers are visible. Gastric ulcers are another name for them when they develop inside your stomach. Duodenal ulcers are the name for when they occur in the top portion of your small intestine.

Some individuals may not even be aware they have an ulcer. Heartburn and stomach pain are among the symptoms experienced by others. If an ulcer ruptures or starts to bleed heavily, it can become quite deadly (also known as a hemorrhage).

Not all ulcers result in symptoms. Symptoms are only present in around 25% of ulcer patients. Several of these signs include:

Abdomen ache

Burp, bloating, or a sense of fullness

Heartburn

Nausea \svomiting

Each person's symptoms might be a little different.

Sometimes having a meal might make the ache go away.

Others find that eating worsens their circumstances.

REFRACTORY ULCER

Refractory peptic ulcer: A refractory peptic ulcer is a larger-diameter ulcer that has been endoscopically verified yet does not heal after 8 to 12 weeks of proton pump inhibitor therapy.

Acid suppression cures >90% of peptic ulcers when nonsteroidal antiinflammatory medication use is discontinued. However, 12 weeks of antisecretory therapy with a proton pump inhibitor are ineffective for about 5 to 10% of ulcers (PPI). Depending on whether Helicobacter pylori has been appropriately eliminated, 5 to 30% of peptic ulcers return during the first year, even with continuing PPI use.

STRESS ULCER

Different situations might cause stress. There are two types of stress: mental or psychological anxiety and physical stress. The likelihood that different kinds of ulcers will be affected by different types of stress may vary. The medical community is divided regarding the actual contribution that mental or psychological stress makes to ulcers of any kind. Many trials and studies have not provided a definitive response to this topic.

However, the study continues as it becomes more apparent that the stomach and brain interact with one another on several different levels. There is also continuing research into how stress affects the body's immune system, which may impact recovery.

It is thought that physical stress initiates the sort of ulcer typically referred to as a stress ulcer. The following are some ways that physical stress may manifest itself:

A significant long-term condition requiring surgery

Severe burns that cause damage to the central nervous system or brain trauma.

Other ulcers, such as peptic and oral ulcers, might not be specifically brought on by stress. There is, however, some data that suggests that emotional stress may make them worse.

The stress brought on by the ulcer is a further connection between pressure and ulcers.

Due to the discomfort and its implications on speaking, chewing, eating, and drinking, mouth ulcers can be very unpleasant and anxious. This social tension exacerbates any mental stress you may already feel.

Due to the possible symptoms they can produce, peptic ulcers can be problematic. They could also make you worry that you won't do anything to aggravate your condition anymore.

Chapter 4

TREATMENT OF STOMACH ULCER

Diagnoses

The health care provider will inquire about your medical history, your symptoms, and the medications you use to determine whether you have a peptic ulcer.

Mention any over-the-counter medications you take, particularly non-steroidal anti-inflammatory drugs (NSAIDs), such as;

→ Aspirin

→ Ibuprofen

→ Naproxen

→ Physique Checkup

A physical examination could aid a clinician in identifying a peptic ulcer. In a physical exam, a doctor will typically.

Examines your belly for signs of bloating uses a stethoscope to listen to the sounds inside your abdomen and taps on it to feel for any soreness or pain.

A blood test entails having a sample of your blood drawn at a lab or your doctor's office. A medical expert analyzes the blood sample to determine whether the findings are within the normal range for various illnesses or infections.

Breathe test for urea. In preparation for a urea breath test, you will consume a special liquid containing urea, a waste product created by your body when it breaks down protein. If H. pylori are present, the bacteria will convert this waste into a harmless gas called carbon dioxide. When you exhale, carbon dioxide usually enters your breath.

At the laboratory, a medical practitioner will collect a sample of your breath by having you inhale it into a bag. Then, they send a sample of your breath to a laboratory for analysis. You have H. pylori in your stomach or small intestine if the carbon dioxide levels in a sample of your breath are greater than usual.

Stool test. To examine a sample of your stool, doctors do a stool test. You will receive a container from your doctor to collect and store your feces at home. You give the sample back to the physician or a business establishment, who then sends it to a lab for examination. H. pylori can be detected in stool samples.

Biopsy and upper gastrointestinal (GI) endoscopy

An endoscope is used by a gastroenterologist, surgeon, or other qualified healthcare providers to view your upper GI tract during an upper GI endoscopy. Both a hospital and an outpatient facility are where this treatment is performed.

To administer a sedative an intravenous (IV) needle will be inserted into your arm. During the surgery, sedatives might keep you comfortable and at ease. The surgery can occasionally be carried out without sedation. You will be given a liquid anesthetic to gargle or spray on the back of your throat. The physician will gently insert the endoscope into the duodenum, stomach, and esophagus. The lining of your upper gastrointestinal system can be closely inspected thanks to a tiny camera attached to the endoscope that transmits a video image to a monitor. The endoscope makes your stomach and duodenum more visible by pumping air into them.

GI upper series

Your upper GI tract's shape is examined during an upper GI series. This test is carried out by an x-ray technician in a hospital or an outpatient facility. The x-ray images are read and reported on by a radiologist. There is no need for an anesthetic. A medical specialist will advise you on preparing for the surgery, including when to cease eating and drinking.

The patient will stand or sit before an x-ray machine during the process and consume the chalky liquid barium. Your esophagus, stomach, and small intestine are coated with barium so your doctor can more clearly view the contours of these organs on x-rays.

Following the test, you could experience bloating and nausea for a short while. You can have white or light-colored barium stools for a few days following that. You'll receive guidance from a medical practitioner regarding what to eat and drink following the test.

X-rays and computer technology are combined in a CT scan to produce the images. A medical expert may administer a solution for you to drink along with an injection of contrast medium, a specialized dye. You will be placed on a table that glides into an x-ray machine with the shape of a tunnel. In a hospital or outpatient facility, an x-ray technician performs the process, and a radiologist interprets the pictures. There is no need for an anesthetic.

A peptic ulcer that has damaged the wall of your stomach or small intestine can be identified via a CT scan. X-rays and computer technology are combined in a CT scan to produce the images. A medical expert may administer a solution for you to drink along with an injection of contrast medium, a specialized dye. You will be placed on a table that glides into an x-ray machine with the shape of a tunnel. In a hospital or outpatient facility, an x-ray technician performs the process, and a radiologist interprets the pictures. There is no need for an anesthetic.

A peptic ulcer that has damaged the wall of your stomach or small intestine can be identified via a CT scan.

Conventional treatment of ulcer

Proton pump inhibitors (PPIs) and histamine-2 (H2) receptor antagonists, two standard therapies for peptic ulcers, have been shown to cause side effects, relapses, and a variety of pharmacological interactions. On the other hand, medicinal plants and the chemical compounds they produce can be used to cure and prevent a wide variety of illnesses.

Antibiotics: Antibiotics can treat an ulcer if the H. pylori bacteria are the cause. Typically, the physician may recommend triple or quadruple therapy, which combines several antibiotics with medications for heartburn.

Triple treatment: Combining two antibiotics, such as amoxicillin and clarithromycin, plus a proton pump inhibitor is a triple treatment. The doctor can replace metronidazole (Flagyl) with amoxicillin if you have a penicillin allergy. The best treatment is quadruple therapy, which consists of two antibiotics (metronidazole and tetracycline), bismuth, and a proton-pump inhibitor. This approach is recommended if you have previously used these antibiotics or reside in a region with metronidazole or clarithromycin resistance. Whatever the strategy, you must take all pills for 10 to 14 days.

Inhibitors Pressure pump: PPIs prevent further harm to the ulcer as it heals naturally by lowering the amount of acid your stomach generates. Typically, they are recommended for 4 to 8 weeks.

H2 inhibitors: These drugs are also known as H2-receptor antagonists or histamine receptor blockers.

They prevent the natural chemical histamine from telling your stomach to produce acid. Cimetidine (Tagamet), famotidine (Pepcid), and nizatidine are examples of H2 blockers (Axid).

Bismuth: This drug covers the ulcer, which also shields it from stomach acid. Infections with H. pylori may also be eliminated by it. It is typically prescribed by doctors together with antibiotics.

Antacids: They don't treat ulcers; they may temporarily lessen your discomfort. Antibiotics may also stop functioning if you take an antacid. Before taking an antacid for peptic ulcer disease, consult your doctor

The most frequently used PPIs to treat stomach ulcers include omeprazole, pantoprazole, and lansoprazole.

Although they often have minor side effects, these can include:

Headaches

Constipation or diarrhea, nausea, headache, dizziness, and rashes

Once the course of treatment is over, these should disappear.

Your doctor could advise surgery if you have a terrible ulcer that keeps returning and doesn't get better with medicines.

Surgery: If you have a bleeding ulcer, you'll require immediate surgery (also called a hemorrhaging ulcer). The surgeon will locate and treat the bleeding source, typically a tiny artery at the ulcer's base. To repair holes in the stomach or duodenal wall, a perforated ulcer, or both, you'll require surgery (the first part of your small intestine).

Some patients choose surgery to reduce the quantity of stomach acid their bodies produce. Talk in-depth about the potential drawbacks with your doctor before you do that. Your ulcer may recur, affect your liver, or experience "dumping syndrome," which results in persistent abdominal pain, diarrhea, vomiting, or sweating after eating.

NATURAL REMEDY TREATMENT

There are numerous natural treatment alternatives that could aid in the treatment or prevention of stomach ulcers.

Fruits, vegetables, and other plant-based products include flavonoids, which have natural anti-inflammatory and antioxidant qualities. They may reduce ulcer-related inflammation and guard against NSAID damage to the lining of the stomach wall.

Foods high in flavonoids include

→ Berries

→ Tea with apples

→ Onions

→ Soy tomatoes, broccoli, Brussels sprouts, and

→ Carrots

→ Vitamin E

A type of naturally occurring fat-soluble vitamin is vitamin E. It can lessen the production of peroxided lipids inside the human body and safeguard the oxidized substances. Additionally, it has the ability to improve skin quality, and treat climacteric syndrome and male sterility. It can also speed up hormone secretion. Even the eye's lens's peroxidation can be controlled to increase blood flow and prevent myopia. Medical study has shown a direct correlation between altered fat peroxidation and the gastric mucous membrane's poor immunity. Vitamin E controls how fat is oxidized, eliminates free radicals, and safeguards cells. Additionally, it can enhance blood circulation, increase oxygen delivery, and speed up capillary and tiny blood vessel hyperplasia, all of which can help an ulcer heal more quickly. Additionally, it can halt the growth of Helicobacter pylori to stop ulcers from returning. Vegetables, nuts, lean meat, and eggs are rich sources of vitamins. For instance, both spinach and cabbage are rich sources of vitamin E. People can therefore increase their daily intake of these items to the greatest extent possible. As a result, gastrointestinal ulcers can be effectively treated, and several other bodily issues can also be resolved.

Bananas

The effectiveness of Musa sapientum pulp as a component of herbal medicine has been examined and confirmed. According to specific research, green bananas' pectin and phosphatidylcholine help to reinforce the mucous-phospholipid barrier that shields the gastrointestinal mucosa. Leucocyanidin, a naturally occurring flavonoid derived from the unripe banana (Musa sapientum) pulp, has been shown in other investigations to protect gastric mucosa from erosions. By thickening gastric mucus, leucocyanidin and its synthetic counterparts, hydroxymethylated leucocyanidin, and tetra-allyl leucocyanidin were reported to protect the stomach mucosa in rat models of aspirin-induced erosions. Other research also shows that banana pulp powder has anti-ulcerogenic properties against aspirin, indomethacin, phenylbutazone, prednisolone, and cysteamine- and histamine-induced duodenal ulcers in rats and guinea pigs, respectively.

A regular meal for the inhabitants of South-Western Nigeria is yam flour, which is combined with dried Musa sapientumpeels. According to folklore, this meal can help patients with ulcers and gastrointestinal pain.

Honey

Although you may have used honey to treat cold symptoms in the past, it is capable of much more. According to studies, honey can combat germs and fungi in the body because it has antibacterial and antifungal qualities. Additionally, it possesses antioxidant and antiviral effects. GI inflammation has been treated with honey in the past.

Ginger

People have used spice ginger for many years to soothe upset stomachs. A study examining ginger's impact on inflammatory bowel disease discovered that it could target intestinal inflammation and prevent harm. Additionally, it encouraged gut-healing components.

Additionally, studies have indicated ginger can help prevent stomach ulcers by H. pylori, stress, alcohol, and NSAIDs.

Cabbage

Antioxidants, chemicals that lessen cell damage from free radicals, are abundant in cabbage juice. Inflammation and sickness may develop in your body if free radicals build up (3Trusted Source).

Vitamin C, a substance with numerous critical functions in the body, is particularly abundant in cabbage. Additionally to promoting immunological function, vitamin C is a potent antioxidant.

Anthocyanins are abundant in red cabbage. These plant pigments, which also have potent antioxidant capabilities, give red cabbage its reddish-purple color. Diets high in anthocyanins have various advantages, including a lower risk of heart disease (5Trusted Source).

In addition, some of the antioxidants in cabbage juice might be anti-cancer. According to a test-tube study, cabbage juice caused human breast cancer cells to die. This result was linked to the juice's high quantity of indoles, an antioxidant.

Garlic

Antioxidant and antibacterial properties are present in garlic. According to a study, consuming a garlic supplement can reduce the likelihood of H. pylori colonizing the G.I tract, which reduces the risk of developing stomach ulcers. The body's inflammation is also reduced by garlic.

Capsaicin

Recent research has revealed that the primary cause of gastric ulcers, one of the most prevalent illnesses affecting people, is a stomach infection with the bacteria Helicobacter Pylori. Additionally, excessive stomach acid output, a decrease in gastric mucosal blood flow, non-steroidal anti-inflammatory medicines (NSAIDs), alcohol, smoking, stress, and other factors are contributing to the development of ulcers.

It is a belief among some segments of the people in this nation and possibly elsewhere that "red pepper," also known as "Chilli," a common spice ingested in large quantities, causes "gastric ulcers" due to its irritating and possibly acid-secreting nature. It is advised to either limit or prevents its use for those who have ulcers. However, new research has shown that the primary ingredient in chilies, "capsaicin," is not what causes ulcers to form but rather a "benefactor.

Although it does not stimulate, capsaicin inhibits the production of acid and increases the production of alkali, mucus secretions, and especially stomach mucosal blood flow, which aids in the prevention and treatment of ulcers. Capsaicin works by igniting the stomach's afferent neurons, which provide signals for defense against harm-causing substances. Gastric ulcers are 3 times more common in "Chinese" people than in Malaysians and Indians, who tend to consume more chilies, according to epidemiologic surveys conducted in Singapore. How long does stomach ulcer take to heal?

Soon after you stop taking a medicine that produces an ulcer, the ulcer should start to heal. An anti-acid medication can help with healing and pain relief for two to six weeks.

After the H. pylori bacteria are eliminated, the ulcers they created can heal. Usually, you will take acid-suppressing medication for two weeks while also taking antibiotics. After then, you might continue taking acid-suppressing medicine for four to eight more weeks.

Compared to duodenal ulcers, gastric ulcers usually heal more slowly. It can take up to two or three months for uncomplicated stomach ulcers to fully recover. It usually takes six weeks for duodenal ulcers to heal.

Antibiotics are not always necessary to treat an ulcer. If the bacteria are not eliminated, an ulcer may return, or another ulcer may develop close by.

CHAPTER 5

DIET FOR STOMACH

Foods high in antioxidants may be helpful if an H. pylori infection is the root cause of your stomach ulcer. They might support you in defending yourself, boosting your immune system, and battling the disease. They might also aid in preventing stomach cancer.

Antioxidant-rich foods include blueberries, cherries, and bell peppers. Calcium and B vitamins are found in leafy greens like kale and spinach.

Sulforaphane, a substance found in broccoli, has anti-H. Pylori properties. According to certain studies, olive oil's fatty acids can assist in treating an H. pylori infection.

Clinical trials have shown promise for fermented probiotic meals. Trusted source for treating ulcers. These foods, such as kimchi, miso, and sauerkraut, may stop an infection from returning.

Additionally, turmeric is also being researched as a potential ulcer therapy.

Onion, licorice, and decaffeinated green tea complete the list of foods you may want to include in your diet. Other food items include;

→ Cauliflower

→ Apples

→ Raspberries

→ Blackberries

→ Strawberries

→ Cherries

→ Peppers, Bell

→ Carrots

→ Broccoli

→ Greens with leaves, like kale and spinach

→ Foods high in probiotics, such as kombucha, miso, sauerkraut, kefir, and yogurt.

→ Olive oil and other oils made from plants

→ Green tea without caffeine, licorice, honey, garlic, and turmeric.

→ Supplement maybe beneficial

Antibiotics are frequently used to treat H. pylori-related peptic ulcers. Probiotics, cranberries, melatonin, lactoferrin, berberine, and licorice are a few supplements that may help eradicate H. pylori or lessen the adverse effects of antibiotics used to treat it.

BENEFITS OF STOMACH ULCER DIETS

An ulcer diet aims to ease the discomfort and irritability caused by peptic ulcers, which are painful lesions on the lining of your stomach, esophagus, or small intestine.

Ulcers are not brought on by or treated by food or drink. But although some meals aggravate ulcers and jeopardize the built-in defenses of your digestive tract, others aid in the regeneration of damaged tissue.

CHAPTER 6

BLEEDING ULCER- WHY IT IS THE MOST DANGEROUS TYPE OF ULCER

Your digestive tract may get blocked by an untreated ulcer that becomes infected or scars. It can infect your abdominal cavity by puncturing your stomach or small intestine. Peritonitis is a condition brought on by that.

Anemia, bloody vomit, or bloody stools can result from bleeding ulcers. Hospitalization is frequently required for a bleeding ulcer. Life-threatening internal hemorrhage is present. Surgery can be necessary if there is a perforation or significant bleeding.

THE SYMPTOMS OF BLEEDING ULCER

Vomiting blood, which may appear red or black, or vomiting blood.

Having blood in the feces or having tarry or black stools

Difficulty breathing

Feeling weak

Nausea or diarrhea

Unaccounted-for weight loss

The appetite shifts

CONCLUSION

The American College of Gastroenterology, a group of medical professionals with expertise in the digestive system, claims that there is no particular diet that someone with ulcers needs to adhere to. Ulcers are neither caused nor exacerbated by dietary decisions.

The basis for current dietary advice is discovering that Helicobacter pylori, a significant contributor to ulcers, may be combated by particular foods' contents.

While peptic ulcers are the most prevalent type, there are numerous other varieties, many of which are brought on by underlying diseases. The etiology of an ulcer will determine how to treat it.

There are over-the-counter remedies that might lessen

the discomfort that ulcers might cause. The sooner you

discuss your symptoms with your doctor, the sooner you

might be able to get relief.

REFERENCE

→ https://www.mountsinai.org/health-library/diseases-conditions/peptic-ulcer

→ https://www.nhs.uk/conditions/stomach-ulcer/

→ https://www.healthline.com/health/bleeding-ulcer

→ https://www.healthline.com/health/stomach-ulcer

→ https://www.webmd.com/digestive-disorders/understanding-ulcers-treatment

→ https://my.clevelandclinic.org/health/diseases/22314-stomach-peptic-ulcer

→ https://www.mayoclinic.org/diseases-conditions/peptic-ulcer/diagnosis-treatment/drc-20354229

→ https://www.verywellhealth.com/symptoms-of-peptic-ulcer-complications-1742819

→ https://my.clevelandclinic.org/health/diseases/22314-stomach-peptic-ulcer